Bulletproof Diet

Eat Fats, Lose Fats

The information herein is offered for informational purposes solely, and is universal as so. The presentation of the information is without contract or any type of guarantee assurance.

The trademarks that are used are without any consent, and the publication of the trademark is without permission or backing by the trademark owner. All trademarks and brands within this book are for clarifying purposes only and are the owned by the owners themselves, not affiliated with this document.

Table of Contents

Introduction 5

What is the Bulletproof Diet? 7

Intermittent Fasting 11

How to Get Started 18

Food 22

Sustaining Bulletproof 35

Meal Planning Guide 37

Breakfast Recipes 48

Lunch Recipes 53

Dinner Recipes 61

Dessert Recipes 75

Smoothie Recipes 87

Conclusion 95

Introduction

Congratulations on downloading *Bulletproof Diet: Lose Fats, Eat Fats* and thank you for doing so.

In an urbanized city, convenient food has become easily accessible to city dwellers. Most people find themselves unknowingly attached to the quick fix food diet. This leads to the feeling of lethargic, fatigue or unexplained discomfort pains anywhere as a symptom of non-optimized health.

The Bulletproof diet gives the body a wonderful chance to re-optimize and fine-tune for the right clean energy boost. It enables you to eat a wide variety of food so that you do not feel deprived in anyway. Key is mainly how to incorporate addition of some food to your diet, method of food preparation and also the best sequence or timing to consume them.

Imagine this: A happy diet plan that provides you high level of energy throughout the day which you can eat snacks in between meals guilt-free and no itch to over eat at meal times.

This book seeks to help you see through such desirable change and aims to provide you the necessary tools for it to be a sustainable and enjoyable journey. You will uncover the marvels of what the Bulletproof Diet is and how it works by burning fat in the following chapters. Useful pointers are also shared on how to stay Bulletproof while eating out or on vacation. You will also get hot tips on meal planning with sample shopping list included. It is understandable that abrupt diet change is uncomfortable and unsustainable for most people. Hence, there is another chapter that gives you a rundown of what foods to eat, what to test, what to limit, and what to avoid.

In this book, you will find the diet to be categorized into breakfast, lunch, dinner, dessert, and smoothies chapters respectively. These chapters are filled with recipes for you to try and enjoy. Please feel free to tweak the recipes to your personal taste and preference.

Before you get all excited to jump in right away, please be aware also that you should consult professional advice from your doctor or nutritionist especially if you have any health issues or dietary restrictions prior any big diet change.

Once you have cleared that, let us get started on the amazing life changing experience!

What is the Bulletproof Diet?

The Bulletproof Diet encourages you to find and avoid food sensitivities. It helps you avoid toxins that keep you from being the real you.

The founder of the Bulletproof Diet, Dave Asprey didn't stumble upon this way of life. He spent years monitoring his health to find the hidden components that were changing the way he performed, felt, looked, his happiness and relationships. After getting the results, he used smart drugs to get his brain back on. He added supplements. He experimented with numerous diets to find out what worked, what didn't work and why it worked. He found out that toxins, gut bacteria, inflammation, neurotransmitters, hormones and numerous other factors play different roles in your body. They all effect your body when it comes to energy levels, hunger, and even weight loss. He gave the findings to family and friends and watched them lose weight fast as well. They also increased their willpower and mental focus. The trick is reducing your body's response by eating less food with anti-nutrients like mycotoxins, mold toxins, oxalates, phytates, and lectins. By avoiding the foods that turn on your immune system, and eating the foods that create healthy gut bacteria, you will keep yourself healthier.

How the Bulletproof Diet Works?

The Bulletproof Diet lets you know what to eat and how much to eat on top of how to cook it and when to eat. The diet is founded on tons of organic vegetables, a moderate amount of good protein, and large amounts of healthy fats to be eaten at just the right time that will create incredible levels of weight loss and energy.

The roadmap shows you how to pick foods that give the most energy and vitamins. These foods contain the smallest amount of inflammation-causing, performance robbing toxins and anti-nutrients.

With the right food fed into our body system, it directly translates to a clearer and happier state of mind which cascades also to a more positive social-emotional aura.

By targeting 50 to 60 percent of your calories from healthy fats that are easy and tastes great, 20 percent from proteins, and vegetables making up the rest.

By eating foods in the green zone, you can just sit back and watch the miracle happen. There is no need to count calories, no need to measure your food. You should eat until you are full and be happy with the benefits of consuming good food. You will soon start to feel your hormones, body, and brain wake up. You will lose weight effortlessly and gain muscle mass with no or very little exercise.

This diet may look like the caveman, primal, or paleo diets because of what our ancestors might have eaten. There are similarities but this diet's nutritional approach is a little bit different from the paleo-style diets. This diet came from researching human performance and biochemistry. It doesn't ignore supplements because the cavemen didn't. It also doesn't uphold the foods our ancestors ate. The Bulletproof Diet fixes the problems that come up from eating the paleo diet for a long time.

Why Bulletproof Diet Works for You?

The bulletproof diet claims to reduce the risks for seasonal allergies, obesity, overweight, migraine headaches, insulin sensitivity, inflammation, high triglycerides, Hashimoto's disease, gout, food cravings, diabetes, cardiovascular disease, certain cancers, brain fog, and acne.

The diet lets you lose weight with no hunger and no cravings. You will be able to have your brain at full power every day all day long. Your newfound willpower and energy will be beyond your wildest dreams.

Most other diets may have certain rules that can cause you to feel guilty or deprived if you don't do exactly everything the diet says. That can cause a negative relationship with you and food. Furthermore, it can also cause you to have binges and crashes.

Diets that make you feel guilty or are restrictive are not feasible. Bulletproof diet works by showing the recommended food on an umbrella. It does not matter if you are getting the most benefits from eating nutrient-dense, anti-inflammatory foods from the green region. Or if you are having foods in the region that need to be tested and be eaten once a while from the yellow zone. Or consuming foods that are terribly bad for you from the red zone. You will know how each food will affect and make you feel.

Most people feel that they are at their best when they eat foods from the green zone. Just knowing that you don't have to consume the same foods every single day will make it easier for you to succeed. The diet focuses on creating a functional body that is strong. Losing weight literally is a side effect that will happen when your body is working like a well-oiled machine.

As with any diet, check with your doctor before you start a new diet. This diet is not to be used as a replacement for any professional diagnosis or for the treatment of any medical conditions.

Intermittent Fasting

Intermittent fasting is a pattern of eating and not a diet. It helps you schedule your meals in a way that gives you the most use. Intermittent fasting changes when you eat not what you eat.

Why does it help you to change the time that you eat?

The first thing is that it will make you lean. You don't have to do a weird diet or cut your calories. In fact, you keep the calories you eat the same. Some people even eat more during a short timeframe. You will notice that you will become leaner but with a muscle mass loss.

Losing weight is the reason most people fast. It is also the simplest way we can take off bad weight and keep on the good weight because it doesn't require any changes to our behavior. This is great because it reflects that it is simple enough to take actions but significant enough to make an observable difference.

To know the reason on intermittent fasting helps in fat loss, you must see the difference between your state when fasting and your state when you are fed.

Fed state is when you body is absorbing and digesting your food. The start of your fed state is when you consume food, and will continue 3-5 hours until your body has completely digested and absorbed your food. It is hard for your body to get rid of fat while you are in the fed state because the insulin levels are too high.

Once that timespan is over, you enter the absorptive state; this is just a fancy way of say that your body isn't absorbing food. This state will continue for 8-12 hours after all your food has been absorbed. After this you will enter the fast state. Your insulin levels are low during this state, and therefore you burn more fat.

Fat that you couldn't burn at any other time can be burned during the fasted state.

It takes 12 hours after we have eaten for our bodies to enter the fasted state. It is very rare that we get in to this state. This is the main reason most people who do the intermittent fasting, could lose fat without changing any other areas of their life. Fasting put your body into a state that burns fat that we normally don't get to with a normal eating schedule.

Intermittent Fasting Benefits

Sure, it's great that you will lose fat, but that shouldn't be the only reason for you to try fasting. There are many positive benefits below that you can gain out of it.

1. Improve your life longevity

Numerous studies have shown that rodents that feast one day and fast the following day often take in lower calories overall than they would normally and they live just as long as other rodents eating calorie-restricted meals daily.

In a 2003 study overseen by Mark Mattson, head of the National Institute on Aging's neuroscience laboratory, rodents that fasted regularly were healthier by some measures than rodents subjected to continuous calorie restriction. Results shown that the rodents on intermittent fasting had lower levels of insulin and glucose in their blood which signified increased sensitivity to insulin and a reduced risk of diabetes.

Hence, scientists have long discovered over time that decreasing calories can help lengthen life. It implies that human bodies will always find ways to survive when in starving mode.

Intermittent fasting will activate the same mechanics to extend life just like restricting calories. You will get the benefits of having a long life and not having to starve yourself.

2. Gives you a simpler day.

We all need to reduce stress, have a simpler life, change our behavior. Intermittent fasting provides added simplicity to our lives. When you wake up, there's no need to worry about breakfast, you grab a cup of Bulletproof coffee with 2 tsp butter and start your day.

We all like to eat and most of us like to cook, so eating three meals is never a hassle. Intermittent fasting allows us to eat one fewer meal. We don't have to stress about, cook, or plan one more meal. It just makes our lives simpler and we all like that.

3. May reduce cancer risks.

There have been debates on this. There aren't many experiments performed to clearly define the relationship of fasting and cancer. According to some early reports things are starting looking positive.

A study of 10 cancer patients showed that fasting before chemotherapy lessened the effect. This also supports a different study with cancer patients that used the alternate day fasting method. They stated that when a patient fasted before chemotherapy could result in fewer deaths and more cure rates.

The comparison of different studies about disease and fasting have suggested that fasting just doesn't reduce the chance of getting cardiovascular disease and cancer.

4. It's easy.

Most diets fail because of the wrong food choices. People tend not to follow diets all the way through. It's not a nutritional problem just behavior problem.

Intermittent fasting is easy once you realize you don't have to continually eat. A study showed that obese adults had a great response to intermittent fasting. They people involved even took to it quickly.

Diets seem easy to think about but challenging to follow through. However, it is the complete opposite with intermittent fasting. It can be hard to think about, but it is rather simple to do.

All of us think about going on a diet some time or other. We even find a diet we want to try and its looks like a breeze. Once we get into it, it starts becoming tough. If you are used to a low-carb diet thinking about going to a diet low in fat seems easy. You would get to have all the carbs you wanted like bananas, corn, potatoes, jelly, bread, bagels and they all sound appealing. But if you were to really follow a diet low in fat you would quickly grow tired of the diet and you would only end up longing for bacon. This goes to show, it's easy to think about diets, but following through with them is hard.

Intermittent fasting might be different thing to think about. You may be thinking how can you not eat for 24 hours. You may also be thinking that you could never do that. Once you start, it's easy. You don't have to worry about where to eat or what to eat for at least one of your daily meals. It is very liberating. The amount of money you spend of food will go down drastically. You will realize that you don't even feel hungry. It is unimaginable to realize that you don't always have to have food. Once you start doing it, it becomes seemingly easy.

As intermittent fasting is so manageable, there is no reason you should not try it. It gives a large list of health benefits without making you do a big lifestyle change.

If fasting sounds like something you want to try, here are some options for you.

Daily Fasting

The time that you start your six hours eating time is completely up to you. You could choose to eat from 6 am to noon, or you could eat from 8 until 2 pm. You pick what works best for you.

Daily fasting, of course, is done daily but it causes it to become easier to get into the habit. You've probably never realized that you naturally eat at the same time every day. Fasting is the same thing, you just aren't eating at certain times.

The disadvantage of this is you aren't getting the same number of calories by just eating a couple of meals like you would with more meals. It is hard to make yourself eat larger meals and a regular basis. Many people who try fasting will lose weight. This can be good or bad. It just depends on your goals.

Weekly Fasting

The easiest way to start fasting is by trying it once a week or even just once a month. Occasional fasting gives you many of the same benefits we have already discussed, so if it's not just for cutting calories there are still health benefits.

Like, lunch on Monday is going to be your final meal of the day. Then you will go without eating until lunch on Tuesday. You will still be eating every day, but you will still be fasting for 24 hours a day. This way you may not lose weight because you are only cutting out two meals a week. If you want to bulk up or keep weight on, this is a good option.

There are several variations to make it work for you. When you travel for a long time, or you have consumed a large meal, then you would greatly benefit from a 24 hour fast.

The most helpful thing of fasting for 24 hours, is moving past the thought of fasting. When you fast for the first time, you will soon realize you aren't going to die when you go without food.

Alternate Day

This option will give you more time between fasts.

You would eat dinner on Monday then you wouldn't eat again until Tuesday evening. Then you would eat all day Wednesday, and then start your next fast after dinner on Wednesday.

This fasting style is used in research studies, but it's not the best option in real life.

The added benefit of alternate day fasting is that you have a longer time in the fasting state. This will increase all benefits you get from doing fasting.

You need to be sure that you are eating enough with this type of fasting. On days you get to eat, make sure you eat enough to help your body sustain itself. You need to train yourself to eat more. Learning to have a feast every day of the week will take some planning, consistent eating, and a lot of cooking. The result will be that people who do intermittent fasting will lose weight due to the size of their meals are the same even if you are cutting out a few meals every week.

If you goal is to lose weight, then there shouldn't be much problem. It is rather simple to follow the weekly or daily if you want to maintain your current weight. If you choose to fast for 24 hours several days a week, it may become difficult to eat what you need to on your eating days.

How to Get Started

Any change can be hard. From trying a new restaurant to learning to eat different foods. It doesn't matter if you are trying to lose weight, feel great, or just want to kick ass. It gets worse when you don't even know how to start. I'm about to make is easier for you. It would be better to do the steps in order but don't be too hard on yourself if you can't.

Most people feel like if they don't eat perfect that they have failed. So they just decide to quit. This is a very bad idea. The good thing about this diet is that you don't have to do it verbatim.

The Bulletproof Diet is uniquely different from any of the other diets out there. There are a lot of questions asking if you don't follow the principles and eat vegetables that aren't organic, or the right meat and seafood will it still work. The answer is simply yes. The more that you can do right, the better off you will be.

You can be stronger and healthier by making the slightest changes. For some, it might be to make a check list to go by. You will be shown a guide to change from an ordinary diet to the Bulletproof diet. Changes like exercise will not be included in this guide as this guide will be focused mainly on eating habits. An overload of information can be a problem when you are trying to deal with a job, your family, and even things that make living fun. Thus, we will be looking at diet alterations as the first step.

The steps are accumulative meaning the more you can do, the better you'll become. Take the first step and move forward. It can be a bit scary trying to decide what to eat with all the information out there.

14 Primary Steps Achieving the Bulletproof Diet

1. Cut out sugar. This includes fruit juices and any drinks that contain agave, honey, and high fructose corn syrup.

2. Get calories from healthy fats. Use ghee, coconut oil, Upgraded XCT oil, grass-fed butter, or Brain Octane.

3. Get rid of all gluten. This referring to pasta, cereal, and bread. Don't eat gluten free junk food, either.

4. Get rid of vegetable oil, grain derived oil, and grains in general. This includes canola, soy, and corn. Get rid of all polyunsaturated oils like peanut oil, flax, and walnut.

5. Stop eating synthetic flavorings, colorings, and additives. This means artificial flavorings, dyes, MSG, and aspartame.

6. Eat large amounts of grass-fed meats from animals like bison, lamb, and beef. You can eat this with shellfish, eggs, and fish.

7. Get rid of legumes like lentils, beans, and peanuts. If you absolutely need to consume them, take the steps to soak them, ferment them, and cook them before consumption.

8. Stop consuming pasteurized, homogenized, and processed dairy. High fat foods are okay to be pasteurized, but make sure they are grass-fed. Whole, raw, full fat dairy from grass-fed cows can be feasible for some.

9. Start eating wild seafood and grass-fed meat. Eat free range eggs and duck, turkey, chicken, and pork.

10. Eat only organic vegetables and fruits.

11. Cook gently, if at all. Use water while cooking if possible and use very low temperatures. Absolutely no frying or microwaving.

12. Don't eat more than one or two servings of fruit a day. Eat only low fructose fruits such as lemons or berries instead of apples and watermelon.

13. Use spices. Herb spices like rosemary and thyme over powders. Use only high quality spices that have only been recently opened.

14. Enjoy what you eat!

Some Key Points to Keep in Mind

➢ If you absolutely must eat any type of fake, junk, cheat food, just do it. Don't beat yourself up and think you've failed. The more you go away from the Bulletproof Diet, the less you'll get. The more you do, the more you'll get. Variations are okay and it does not mean that you have failed.

➢ If you start experiencing any sort of acne, allergy, or other side effect after eating dairy, use only ghee as your dairy source. Eat coconut oil and animal fat.

➢ Don't count calories to try to lose weight. Eat until full and stop.

➢ Don't snack. Intermittent fasting is supported, but not mandatory.

➤ Limiting your intake of fruit to one to two servings will help you avoid high triglycerides. The other reasons to limit your consumption won't kill you.

➤ Healthy high fat intake is needed. You need to try to eat 10 to 30 % protein, 5 to 30 % carbohydrate, and 50 to 80 % fat.

➤ Eat the smallest amounts of polyunsaturated fat that you can find. Use supplements like krill and fish oil if you don't eat salmon weekly.

➤ If you are having a hard time finding grass-fed meats, pick the leanest grain-fed meat. When buying grass-fed meat get the fattiest cuts.

➤ Don't use the excuse of not having time. It doesn't take that much time to make Bulletproof Coffee and soft boiled eggs. Making your body and mind healthy is not optional. It is a necessity.

If you can do this somewhat right, you'll get a high energy, high performance, low inflammation lifestyle.

Food

The lists that follow will show what foods to eat, what foods to limit, what foods to test, and what foods to avoid.

Foods to Eat

Fats

- The best: Bulletproof Cocoa Butter, Bulletproof Chocolate, Bulletproof medium-chain triglyceride MCT oil, Bulletproof Brain Octane, ghee, sunflower lecithin, virgin coconut oil, avocado oil or avocados, grass-fed animal fat like lard, tallow, bone marrow not poultry fat, krill oil, free range egg yolks, don't eat if you're allergic to eggs.

- Next best: ghee, grass-fed butter, fermented cod liver oil, fish oil

Protein sources

- Clean whey concentrate

- Gelatin

- Hydrolyzed collagen

- Free range eggs

- Grass-fed beef or lamb

- Low mercury fish

Vegetables: *indicates vegetables that need to be cooked

- Buy organic if possible. Do not buy vegetables with brown spots or that are wilted. Frozen are often better than most fresh.

- Best: olives, fennel, cucumber, celery, cauliflower, Brussel sprouts*, broccoli*, bok choy*, avocado, asparagus.

- Next best: zucchini, summer squash, spinach*, radishes, lettuce, kale*, collard greens*, cabbage*

Protein

- Best: Bulletproof CollaGelatin, Bulletproof Collagen Protein, Bulletproof Whey, colostrum, free range gelatin, free range eggs (as long as you aren't allergic and don't eat just the whites), goat, bison, lamb, beef (make sure it is grass-fed and grass-finished)

- Organ meat: joints for soup, bone marrow, tongue, heart, kidneys, liver of fish, goat, lamb, and beef

- Next best: wild trout, wild tilapia, summer flounder, sockeye salmon, sardines, petrale sole, haddock, anchovies. These are all low-mercury fish.

- Shellfish: oysters, mussels, lobster, real crab

Dairy

- Best: colostrum, grass-fed organic butter, grass-fed organic ghee

- Next best: grass-fed cream, nonorganic grass-fed butter or ghee

Legumes, seeds, and nuts

- No legumes

- Best: coconut

Flavorings and spices: *these usually have toxic mold spores. Use high-quality, fresh whenever you can.

- Best: Bulletproof Vanillamax vanilla powder, Bulletproof Chocolate Powder, sea salt, parsley, ginger*, coffee*, cilantro, apple cider vinegar

- Next best: vanilla*, turmeric, thyme, rosemary, oregano, lavender

Sweeteners

- Best: stevia, erythritol, xylitol

- Next best: sugar alcohol, maltitol, sorbitol

Beverages

- Best: Bulletproof coffee made with Bulletproof coffee beans, mineral water in glass bottles, diluted coconut milk (make sure it doesn't have carrageenan, or guar gum, BPA free, remember that light coconut milk has just had water added), yerba mate, high quality green tea

- Next best: green tea, filtered water with lemon or lime

Cooking methods

- Best: lightly heated, raw. Animal proteins should be eaten rare or raw. Grass-fed animals don't have toxins, pathogens, and parasites that grain-fed animals might have.

- Next best: baked in a conventional oven at 320 or lower, UV oven, steamed al dente

- Poached or boiled is okay. Don't do it every day.

Foods to limit

Fruits and starches need to be limited during the whole diet. Suspect foods need to be tested to see if you have certain reaction to them.

Starches

- Eat in the evening. This should be about 5 percent of the daily calorie intake including fruit.

- Best: carrot (cook if you have IBS), yam, sweet potato, butternut squash, pumpkin fresh (not canned)

- Next best: white rice

- Possibly need to test: plantain, taro, cassava

- Least needed to test: green banana flour, Hi-maize starch, plantain flour, potato starch better known as resistant starch powders. Do not use these food ingredients while on the 14-day program. These foods may work for some but there are some who find their healthy gut bacteria feeds better on connective tissue from meat, collagen, and gelatin.

- Need to test: frozen or fresh organic corn on the cob, banana, brown rice, wild rice, black rice

- Most needed to test: Purple or white potatoes

- Might need to test: quinoa, buckwheat, oats. Oats are very bad if you have problems with your digestive system.

Fruits

- Eat in evening. Do not consume any more than 25 grams a day. This is about two apples.

- Buy organic if possible. If organic isn't possible, remove the skin if the fruit has one.

- Do not consume fruits that are beginning to spoil or are damaged.

- Best: raspberries, lime, lemon, cranberries, coconut, blackberries, avocado

- Next best: tangerine, strawberries, pineapple, blueberries

- Least needed to test: pomegranate, grapefruit

- Need to test: plums, pears, peach, orange, nectarine, lychee, kiwifruit, honeydew, figs, cherries, apricot, apples. Do not eat apples in the first two weeks so you can see if you react to them.

- Most needed to test: watermelon, plantain, persimmon, passion fruit, papaya, melons, mango, guava, grapes, fresh dates, bananas

Foods to Test

Try to avoid these while doing the two-week protocol. Test them to see what you can introduce back into the diet. Being suspect doesn't necessarily mean they are bad. It just means that people might have a bad reaction to them. See what your personal reaction is to the food.

Vegetables to test

- Least needed to test: parsley, leeks, scallions or green onions, green beans, carrots, winter squash, butternut squash, artichokes (don't eat if you have a nightshade sensitivity).

- Need to test: garlic, tomatoes, shallots, peppers, peas, onion, eggplant

- Most needed to test: raw spinach, raw kale, raw collards, raw chard, pumpkin, beets

Fats to test

- Least needed to test: extra virgin olive oil, raw macadamias, free range bacon fat, palm kernel oil, palm oil

- Need to test: non-GMO soy lecithin, cashew butter, unheated nut oils

- Most needed to test: grain-fed ghee and butter, free range chicken fat, free range goose fat, free range duck fat

Proteins to test

- You can have turkey, chicken, goose, duck, or pork a couple times a week, but you won't get the same benefit if you just eat grass-fed meat or fish.

- Least needed to test: free range goose and duck, clean whey isolate, free range pork

- Need to test: free range turkey and chicken, factory raised eggs

- Most needed to test: factory raised meat, hemp protein, sprouted legumes, heated whey

Dairy to test

- Least needed to test: yogurt, raw, full-fat, grass-fed, organic milk

- Need to test: grass-fed, organic cream, butter, or nonorganic grass-fed ghee

- Most needed to test: butter that is grain-fed

Legumes, seeds, and nuts

- Most needed to test: walnuts, pecans, macadamia, hazelnuts, chestnuts, cashews, almonds

- Need to test: Brazil nuts, pine nuts, pistachios

- No legumes

Flavorings and spices *These hide mold spores. Use only high quality fresh when you can.

- Least needed to test: prepared mustard that's organic with no additives. Cloves*, cinnamon, all-spice

- Need to test: table salt, onion, mustard seed

- Most needed to test: all vinegars except apple cider, paprika*, nutmeg*, garlic*, conventional chocolate (should be no less than 85 percent dark chocolate), black pepper*

Sweeteners to test

- Least needed to test: raw honey, non-GMO glucose and dextrose

- Need to test: coconut sugar, maple syrup

- Most needed to test: cooked sugar, agave nectar, agave syrup, brown sugar, white sugar

Beverages to test

- Least needed to test: fresh nut milk, high quality herbal teas, unsweet fresh brewed iced tea, water with muddled fruit, tap water with lemon or lime

- Need to test: bottled nut milks, coconut water bottled or boxed, fresh coconut water, no sugar added bottled iced tea, raw milk, kombucha

- Most needed to test: fruit juice, fresh squeezed

- Alcohols to test: Avoid these during the first 14 days. Document your reaction to each after. Drink responsibility. Dry white wine, dry champagne (these are more suspect), whiskey, tequila, gin, vodka

Cooking methods to test

- Least needed to test: lightly grilled but not burned, simmered

- Need to test: slow cooking, sous vide

- Most needed to test: broiled

Foods to Avoid

Processed foods

- Synthetic flavorings

- Processed ingredients, other chemicals, soy protein, monosodium glutamate (MSG)

GMO ingredients

- This is commonly found in soy, potatoes, sugar cane, cottonseed, corn, and canola crops

- Products made with high-fructose corn syrup, and vegetable oils

Vegetables

- Not as bad: corn on the cob

- Worst: soy, mushrooms, canned vegetables, all other types of corn

Fats

- Chemically damaged fats

- Refined vegetable oils

- Not as bad: flaxseed oil, heated oils, heated nuts, vegetable oil, corn oil, cottonseed oil, soy oil, peanut oil, canola oil, sunflower oil, safflower oil, factory chicken fat

- Worst: commercial lard, oils from GMO grains, artificial trans fats, margarine

Protein

- Not as bad: pea protein, rice protein, farmed seafood, high-mercury seafood

- Worst: cooked dairy (not including butter), cheese, chickpeas, beans, legumes, wheat protein, soy foods, soy protein (like soy sauce, natto, miso, tempeh, tofu, soy burgers, soy milk, soy beans)

Dairy

- Not as bad: yogurt, nonorganic milk, fake butter, low-fat milk, skim milk

- Worst: prepared dairy products (like cheese sauce, cheese spread, coffee creamer, American cheese), conventional ice cream, evaporated milk, condensed milk, dairy replacer, factory dairy, powdered milk, all cheese

Seeds and nuts

- Not as bad: chia seed, flaxseed, peanuts

Legumes

- Not as bad: peanuts, lentils, dried beans, most legumes, dried peas, hummus, chickpeas, garbanzo beans, sprouted legumes

- Worst: corn nuts, soy nuts, soy

Starches

- Worst: gluten-free powders, corn starch, potato starch, other grains, millet, processed dried corn products, polenta, corn mash, corn bread, non-organic corn on the cob, conventionally grown corn, pasta, cereal, baked goods, bread, wheat

Fruit

- Not as bad: cantaloupe

- Worst: canned fruit, jelly, jam, fruit leather, dried fruit, raisins

Flavorings and spices

- Not as bad: tofu, tamari, miso, fermented soy

- Worst: artificial seasonings, artificial flavorings, enzyme modified anything, hydrolyzed gluten, broth, bouillon, textured protein TVP, caseinate, yeast, monosodium glutamate MSG, extracts, spice mixes, commercial dressings

Sweeteners

- Not as bad: high-fructose corn syrup, fruit juice concentrate, fructose

- Worst: tagatose, acesulfame potassium aka Ace-K, sucralose aka Splenda, aspartame aka NutraSweet

Beverages

- Not as bad: pasteurized milk

- Worst: sports drink, aspartame drinks, sweetened drinks, soda, diet drinks, packaged juice, soy milk

- Worst alcohols: beer, red wine, white wine

Ways of cooking

- Not as bad: stir fried

- Bad: microwaved, barbecued

- Worst: deep-fried, charred, blackened, burnt

Sustaining Bulletproof

While you are in maintenance mode, you will get better results from staying as closely as possible to the main diet principles. Start the day with Bulletproof Coffee, stick to Intermittent Fasting on most days. Do the fasting once a week and avoid bad foods when you can. The main differences while in maintenance mode is whether to start eating the test foods. This all depends on your reactions to these foods. These are the foods you tested in the 2-week protocol. When you know the food that you are sensitive to, you can go off into the world and make the best choices for you, your body, and your body's performance.

If you would like to, eat more carbs in the evening. If your pants start to get tight, just cut back. You could even have starch in the morning if you wanted to. You know your body is tough and can deal with it.

You can have something besides coffee for breakfast if it makes you feel better so long as you are in maintenance mode. Just remember to do the intermittent fasting occasionally.

You can eat bad food occasionally if you would like to but just remember that you might feel bad for the next day or two. Small changes are fine and doesn't mean you have failed. You will want to try to stick with the diet if you want to make progress on your weight loss. If you stray too far away from the diet, your performance will start to suffer. If this should happen, just go back to the 2-week protocol, and have a refresher course on the principles of the diet.

Here are a few quick tips to help you stay Bulletproof while on vacation or eating away from home.

1. Choose a protein. Either wild caught or grass-fed. If either of these are not available, choose a white meat like turkey or chicken. These are both a low-fat protein. They have less toxin fats that you will digest. Healthy fats that you get from wild caught fish or grass-fed cows are the best source of fat.

2. Choose a vegetable as your side. Steamed preferably to eliminate any unknown oils that may have been used.

3. Choose a fat. This is the main thing to remember. You want 70 percent of your calories to be from healthy fats. Most restaurants won't have brain octane oil, XCT oil, or grass-fed butter. But most do have avocados. Order as much avocado as they will let you have. You could bring your own fat to add to the meal.

Meal Planning Guide

Here are some basic guidelines for your meals.

Proportions

- Fruit and starch should only be 5 percent of your calories. If weight loss is your priority. Try to avoid them most of the time. If not, you can have a small portion every day.

- Vegetables without starch should be 20 percent of your calories. This will make up a large proportion of your plate because vegetables have low calorie count. If vegetables aren't your favorite, you can coat them in grass-fed butter and sea salt.

- Protein sources should be bulletproof and take up 20 percent of your calories.

- The right kind of fat should take up about 50 to 70 percent of your calorie intake.

- If you don't feel like eating, don't make yourself. If you don't meet the daily guidelines, it's no big deal.

- When you are hungry, eat. Stop when you get full. Try your best not to snack if possible.

Breakfast

- Drink 2 cups of hot brewed Bulletproof Coffee. Make sure you only use Bulletproof Upgraded Coffee. These beans are the highest quality with the lowest level of toxins and no mold. Add two tablespoons butter.

Making sure the butter is grass-fed and unsalted. You can also add two tablespoons Brain Octane C8 Medium Chain Triglyceride Oil or any other MCT oil. If you don't have any other choices, you can use coconut oil. You could also add in the highest quality cinnamon, chocolate or vanilla powder. Use hardwood xylitol, erythritol, or stevia to taste.

- If you need to lose a lot of weight, or you are a largely muscled athlete, or a woman, you will benefit from having some form of protein with your Bulletproof Coffee for the first 60 days. It is recommended to blend collagen protein that comes from grass-fed poultry in your Bulletproof Coffee.

- If you are trying to conceive or are pregnant, you shouldn't drink caffeinated coffee. Try the No-Coffee Vanilla Latte recipe (located in Breakfast Recipe chapter) or use lab-tested decaf.

- Once you've done this for 14 days, or what we call maintenance mode, you can eat something besides just having Bulletproof Coffee. It is best to have a combination of fat and protein such as avocado, smoked salmon, and a poached egg. If you just eat protein without fats is better than having carbs or fruits, this may still cause you to have some cravings.

Intermittent Fasting

- Do not eat anything after you have your morning coffee until lunch or possibly later if you don't feel hungry. This allows you the benefit of intermittent fasting but still being able to have breakfast.

- Your eating window is 6 hours long. This gives you an 18-hour fast.

Evening Meal

- Consume a decent amount of Bulletproof carbs. This should be about 30 grams including vegetables. Eat this with your evening meal only. Have a carb refeed day a couple times a week. On these days eat approximately 100 to 150 grams. This should be done on your Bulletproof Protein Fasting days. The amount will depend on how quickly you want to lose weight, your stress level, and your hunger. Eating less carbs every night will bring on weight loss faster.

- Women need more carbs at least 300 grams on refeed days. If you are pregnant you should eat a limited amount of carbs nightly while keeping all the other principles of the Bulletproof Diet.

- Fill up on fat at dinner. This helps you sleep better. You can also add protein right before bed to help you sleep. Don't consume too much meat. This can leave you with a heavy feeling. Use undenatured whey protein concentrate or hydrolyzed grass-fed collagen peptide. You could also eat some raw honey. You can add these to the No-Coffee Vanilla Latte, too.

Bulletproof Protein Fasting

- Once a week, eat no more than 25 grams of protein.

- If you realize that protein fasting is creating muscle loss or other side effects, you can cut back. Instead of not eating protein for a whole day just skip protein for several meals. You can play around with the amount of protein you are consuming on the Bulletproof Protein Fasting days.

Two-week Bulletproof protocol

- Throw out all the bad junk food in your house

- Use the food guide in the prior chapter as a guide. Focus on the Good foods and try to avoid the test foods and bad ingredients

- Have Bulletproof Coffee for breakfast. If you need to lose a bunch of weight or are a woman over 40, or if coffee does not fill you, you can add 25 to 30 grams of protein like grass-fed collagen protein.

- You need to have huge amounts of vegetables for lunch and dinner. Also, eat healthy fats, a moderate amount of protein, and a little bit of starch after and during dinner. Eat both meals during a six-hour window for the intermittent fasting to work. For example, eat lunch at 1pm and have dinner at 7pm.

- One day a week, usually day 6 and 13, follow the Bulletproof Protein Fasting. This means eating 25 grams of protein and 100 to 150 grams of carbohydrates. If you are a woman, you can eat 300 grams of carbohydrates.

Make sure you keep track of which foods you tested that are bad for you. Each person has their own food sensitivities.

You can get a blood panel test from your doctor if you suspect food allergies.

Start this testing during the two-week protocol to see whether any good foods are bad for you specifically.

A shopping list is included here which might make your trip to the grocery store easier. You obviously don't have to get everything. It's just meant to provide you with options. You can choose from the choices in your area.

The foods on the list are either in the green zone or yellow zone if the Bulletproof Diet. They are not in any particular order.

Protein

Muscle Meats

1. Bison

2. Beef

3. Goat

4. Lamb

5. Pork

6. Eggs (no omega-3)

7. Turkey

8. Duck

9. Goose

Seafood

1. Haddock

2. Cod

3. Anchovies

4. Salmon

5. Real crab

6. Mussels

7. Lobster

8. Flounder

9. Oysters

10. Trout

11. Tilapia

Organ meats (make sure these are from grass-fed animals)

1. Heart

2. Liver (fish, goat, lamb, beef)

3. Tongue

4. Kidneys

5. Bone marrow

6. Joints for soup bones

Fats and oils

1. Coconut oil

2. Grass-fed butter

3. Ghee

4. Medium-chain triglycerides oil

5. Coconut flesh

6. Cocoa butter (90% cacao works too)

7. Avocado oil

8. Animal fat and lard (only from grass-fed)

9. Extra virgin olive oil

10. Coconut milk (try to find without guar gum and BPA free)

Leafy Vegetables

1. Bok Choy

2. Spinach

3. Brussel sprouts

4. Parsley

5. Cilantro

6. Collards

7. Cucumber

8. Celery

9. Artichokes

10. Fennel

11. Carrots

Safe Carbs, tubers and roots

1. Sweet potatoes

2. Carrots

3. Yams

4. Winter squash

5. Cassava

6. Rutabaga

7. White rice

Remember it's better to avoid all grains but white rice a few times a week shouldn't hurt.

Fruits

If you want to lose fat, buy berries or other low sugar fruits

1. Limes or lemons

2. Berries like blueberries, cranberries, blackberries, raspberries, strawberries.

3. Tomatoes

4. Melons such as honeydew and cantaloupe

5. Nectarine or peaches

6. Citrus like oranges and grapefruit

Seeds and Nuts

Nuts spoil quickly therefore they are not a low toxin food. Mold is a big issue with nuts. Get raw nuts and freeze the or at least keep them refrigerated. Soaking nuts for 18 hours before eating might reduce some toxins but not mold. Buy nuts in their shell.

1. Almonds

2. Coconut

3. Brazil Nuts

4. Cashews

5. Hazelnuts

6. Pecans

7. Macadamia Nuts

8. Pistachios

9. Chia seeds

10. Pine nuts

Dairy

This one is very easy. Do not change this list.

1. Grass-fed butter like Kerry Gold, Anchor or any other brand you can find that is 100 percent grass-fed.

Flavorings and Spices

Powdered spices can be contaminated with mold. Buy herb/leaf based spices.

1. Himalayan pink salt

2. Apple cider vinegar

3. Ginger

4. Unmodified, pure sea salt

5. Parsley

6. Cilantro

7. Turmeric

8. Oregano

9. Lavender

10. Rosemary

11. Thyme

12. Cinnamon

13. Sage

14. Cloves

15. Allspice

Sweeteners

1. Xylitol

2. Erythritol

3. Stevia

When it comes to buying food, it is best to get it from the person who butchered it. Some places have higher standards than others.

Hopefully this list was helpful.

Breakfast Recipes

Vanilla Latte

Ingredients

- ½ tsp. organic cinnamon plus ¼ tsp. cardamom, or 1 tsp. cocoa powder

- 1 tsp. unsweetened vanilla powder

- 2 Tbsp. MCT Oil

- 2 Tbsp. ghee or grass-fed butter

- 2 cups hot water, filtered

Directions

Put all the ingredients in your blender. Blend until incorporated.

Ultimate Bulletproof Coffee

Ingredients

- 1 Tbsp. grated 90% cacao

- 2 Tbsp. ghee or grass-fed butter

- 1 to 2 Tbsp. Brain Octane oil or XCT oil

- 250 to 300 ml brewed Bulletproof coffee that has been brewed with a pinch of Vanillamax

Directions

Put everything in the blender except the cacao. On high, blend until creamy. Top with grated cacao.

Pumpkin Spice Un-Latte

Ingredients

- ½ tsp. Vanillamax

- 1 tsp. pumpkin pie spice

- 1 Tbsp. butter, grass-fed, unsalted

- 3 Tbsp. pumpkin puree, organic

- 3 Tbsp. Brain Octane Oil

- 1 ¼ cup unsweetened, full fat coconut milk

Optional: 2 Tbsp. whipped coconut cream or raw whipped cream on top

Optional: 1 Tbsp. organic maple syrup or 1 to 2 tsp. xylitol

Directions:

1. Place all ingredients in saucepan. Simmer for 5 minutes over medium heat. Stir well to blend oils and spices.

2. Pour 2 ½ cups coffee, and pumpkin mixture from saucepan into blender. Blend for 30 seconds on high speed until frothy and creamy.

3. An option if you don't have a blender is to add the coffee and pumpkin mixture in a saucepan and blend with an emersion blender. Blend until frothy and smooth.

4. You could also add xylitol to sweeten.

5. You can also top with raw whipped cream on top.

This makes between 4 and 6 cups of coffee. This is not for every day. This is a special treat.

Pumpkin Pancakes

Ingredients

- 1 tsp. VanillaMax
- 1 Tbsp. pumpkin spice
- 2 Tbsp. coconut flour
- ½ cup almond or flax meal
- 1 tsp. baking powder
- 1 Tbsp. maple syrup
- ½ cup pumpkin puree
- 4 large eggs

Directions

1. Mix all ingredients in blender.
2. Grease skillet with ghee or grass-fed butter
3. Place about ¼ cup of batter onto hot skillet. Cook pancakes over low heat until each side is golden and bubbly. This will take about 3 minutes per side.
4. Place butter on top of hot pancakes and sprinkle with vanilla or chocolate collagen bars.
5. Enjoy!

Lunch Recipes

Cauliflower Mash

Ingredients

- ½ tsp. apple cider vinegar

- 2 Tbsp. Brain Octane oil

- 4 Tbsp. unsalted grass-fed butter

- 1 head cauliflower, cut into pieces

- ½ lb. free range, uncured diced bacon

- Sea salt

Directions

1. Lightly cook bacon in large skillet over medium-low heat. Be sure to not let it get crispy and don't let the fat smoke. Set aside and keep the fat in pan.

2. Bring water to boil in pot. Put cauliflower in pot, cover with lid, and allow steam for 15 to 20 minutes.

3. In blender, put ¾ of the head of cauliflower, butter, salt, vinegar, and oil. Blend on high power. Stir in bacon and cauliflower. Pulse until the mixture is chunky.

4. You can add one to two Tbsp. of bacon fat to cauliflower mixture for added flavor.

5. Enjoy!

Sweet Potato Stuffing

Ingredients

- 1 Tbsp. cayenne pepper

- 3 Tbsp. ghee

- 5 diced sweet potatoes

- 3 Tbsp. mixed herbs – Mix equal parts – dried or diced fresh

- Chives

- Rosemary

- Oregano

- Parsley

- Sage

- 2 Tbsp. coconut flour

- Salt

Directions

1. Heat oven to 450.

2. Put diced sweet potatoes in pot and fill with water. Cover and boil. Boil for about 4 minutes or until just tender. Place sweet potatoes in bowl of ice water, cool down slightly and drain well. Make sure you cool off the sweet potatoes here or they won't be crispy later.

3. Place sweet potatoes evenly over a parchment paper lined baking sheet. Don't overcrowd the potatoes. You want to get them crispy.

4. Melt ghee in saucepan and drizzle it over the sweet potatoes. Mix the herbs with cayenne pepper. Sprinkle over the sweet potatoes, and toss to coat them.

5. Add coconut flour and toss again.

6. Bake for 20 minutes or until potatoes get crispy and brown.

Steak Bowl

Ingredients

- 1 tsp. sage
- 1 tsp oregano
- 1 tsp. thyme
- 1 tsp. rosemary
- 1 tsp. parsley
- 1 Tbsp. Himalayan pink sea salt
- 1 tsp. cracked pepper
- 2 Tbsp. extra virgin olive oil
- 1 ½ lb. tri tip
- Brain Octane Oil for drizzling

Directions

1. Heat oven to 350.
2. Trim fat and skin off of the tri tip.
3. Massage extra virgin olive oil onto all sides of meat.
4. Mix spices together to form the herb rub.
5. Rub salt on tri tip then cover with chopped herbs. Make sure it stays on the meat and oil if you need to.

6. Place tri tip on baking sheet and put in oven.

7. Cook for about 20 minutes.

8. Remove meat for oven and allow to rest for around 10 minutes.

9. Slice. Add more salt and drizzle with Brain Octane Oil.

10. Enjoy!

Serve with cauli-rice (the recipe follows) or long-grain rice with lightly sautéed or steamed vegetables.

Lime-Cilantro Cauli-Rice

Ingredients

- 1 scallion, chopped

- Himalayan pink sea salt

- ½ cup fresh cilantro, chopped

- 2 Tbsp. Brain Octane Oil

- 2 Tbsp. butter, unsalted, and grass-fed

- Juice from 1 lime

- 1 cauliflower head

Directions

1.   Place cauliflower in food processor and pulse until it resembles rice.

2.   Melt butter in large saute pan. Add cauliflower. Crowding the pan is fine as it will help the cooking by making a steamy effect. Do not brown the cauliflower. Cook for 5 to 10 minutes, stirring often.

3.   Turn off heat. Add cilantro, oil, and lime juice, and salt to taste. Mix well in pan. Transfer to serving dish. Garnish with scallion.

4.   Enjoy!

Chili Beef Butternut Squash

Ingredients

- 1 butternut squash, cubed

- ¼ tsp. cinnamon

- ½ oz. (2 Tbsp.) grated chocolate bar

- ¼ cup organic tomato paste

- ½ cup gluten-free beer

- ½ cup organic chicken broth

- 2 tsp. basil, dried

- 2 Tbsp. chopped oregano, fresh

- 1 cup water

- 6 medium tomatoes, chopped

- 2 Tbsp. ground cumin

- 1 tsp. cayenne pepper

- 1 tsp. chipotle chili powder

- 2 Tbsp. ancho chili powder

- 1 ½ lb. grass-fed ground beef

- 4 to 5 large garlic cloves, chopped + 1 extra clove chopped and set aside

- 1 cup chopped onion with ¼ cup set aside

- 1 tsp. butter, grass-fed

- 1 Tbsp. XCT Oil

- Salt and pepper to taste

Directions

1. In large skillet, heat butter and oil. Add ¾ cup onion and 4 garlic cloves. Cook on medium heat until the onions become opaque. Add in beef and brown, break into small pieces as it cooks. Season with pepper and salt. Once beef is done add cumin, cayenne, chipotle, and ancho. Stir until combined and set aside.

2. In large saucepan, put the rest of the garlic and onion, water, and chopped tomatoes. Let simmer about 5 minutes on medium heat. Salt lightly. Turn down heat, mix in basil and oregano and simmer a little longer. Add beef and chicken broth. Let simmer about 3 minutes. Add cinnamon and chocolate. Mix together. Let simmer another 5 minutes. Take off heat and cool.

3. Heat oven to 350. Cube butternut squash. Toss with 1 Tbsp. XCT Oil and salt. Place on baking sheet in a single later, and bake it until tender

4. When ready to serve, heat chili over medium heat and add butternut squash.

5. Serve and enjoy!

Dinner Recipes

Spaghetti Squash Bolognese

Ingredients

- 2 Tbsp. butter, grass-fed
- 1 lb. grass-fed beef
- 1 jar organic tomato sauce
- Himalayan sea salt
- Herbs of your choice
- 2 Tbsp. coconut oil
- 1 spaghetti squash

Directions

1. Heat oven to 320.
2. Cut spaghetti squash in half horizontally.
3. Fill baking pan ½ way up with water.
4. Place cut squash on pan with cut side facing up.
5. Put coconut oil and herbs of your choice into the halves.
6. Cover with foil and put in oven.
7. Cook for 30 minutes or until soft enough to scrape

8. While squash is cooking, brown the grass-fed beef in sauce pan.

9. Pour tomato sauce over beef and warm through.

10. Add spices of your choice, again.

11. Once squash has cooled slightly, use fork to scrape the insides of squash to make spaghetti.

12. Pour sauce mixture on top. Top it off with 2 tablespoons butter.

13. Mix sauce and squash.

14. Enjoy!

Turkey and Gravy

Ingredients

- 2 Tbsp. ghee

- 1 – 14 lb. turkey, rinsed, inside and out and patted dry inside and out

Ingredients for Turkey Rub

- 2 tsp. rosemary, finely diced

- 2 tsp. thyme, finely diced

- 1 tsp. sage, finely diced

- ½ tsp. garlic powder

- ½ tsp. onion powder

- 2 tsp. Himalayan pink salt

Ingredients for gravy

- Drippings from turkey

- 3 Tbsp arrowroot powder

- 2 cups free-range turkey or chicken stock

- 2 Tbsp. lemon juice or apple cider vinegar

- Himalayan pink salt

- ½ tsp. garlic powder

Directions

1. Heat oven to 325.

2. Mix spices and herbs to make the rub for turkey.

3. Place turkey in roasting pan. Melt ghee in saucepan and brush over turkey, outside and in.

4. Rub the herb mixture generously over the turkey.

5. Roast turkey for 3 ½ hours. Baste it about every 20 minutes so that is stays moist.

6. Remove the turkey from the roasting pan onto a serving platter and tent with tin foil. Let rest for at least 30 minutes. Do not discard the drippings.

7. To make the gravy, pour the dripping into a saucepan. Place pan over medium heat. Add the arrowroot starch and whisk until the mixture is smooth. Add stock and bring to a boil. Whisk until gravy is smooth. Reduce heat to simmer and continue to cook until gravy is as thick as you want. Add the vinegar and salt. Stir thoroughly.

8. Take off the heat, and serve.

9. Enjoy!

Cranberry Sauce

Ingredients

- ¼ cup xylitol

- Zest from one orange

- ¼ cup water

- 1 lb. frozen cranberries

Directions

Add all ingredients to food processor and pulse until mixture is smooth.

Cassava Egg Rolls

Ingredients for the rolls

- Ghee for frying

- ½ tsp. Himalayan pink sea salt

- ½ cup coconut oil

- 3 cups fresh cassava, boiled and chopped – if finding fresh is too hard, you can substitute 3 cups cassava flour

Ingredients for Filling

- 1 tsp sea salt

- 1 tsp ginger

- 4 Tbsp. garlic coconut aminos

- 1 cup organic shredded carrots

- 2 cups organic red cabbage, shredded

- ½ lb. beef or lamb, grass-fed

Directions

1. Heat oven to 350

2. Bring filtered water to boil in large pot.

3. Peel the cassava root and give it a rough chop.

4. Put chopped cassava in boiling water. Boil for 20 minutes. Done when you can insert a fork in them.

5. Take off heat and drain.

6. Put cassava in blender with sea salt and oil. Blend on high until a consistent, sticky, smooth dough is formed.

7. Line a baking pan with parchment paper. The bigger the pan is the better.

8. Put dough on the parchment paper to cool. Use a rubber spatula, spread dough into a large square. Make it as thin as possible.

9. Cook dough in over for 10 minutes. You don't want to brown it. Just cook it long enough to seal the surface. You need to be able to roll the dough.

10. Prepare the filling while the dough is in the oven. Brown your meat in ghee with salt, coconut aminos, and spices.

11. Remove from heat and let cool. Keep an eye on your dough. Remove when sealed.

12. Get a cast iron skillet ready by adding 2 Tbsp. ghee to skillet, while the dough cools. You may need to add more ghee depending on the size of your skillet.

13. Slice dough into 3 X 3 inch squares, once it is cooled.

14. Put 1 spoonful of filling to your wrapper. Roll and tuck the corner to close all edges.

15. Fry your rolls in the prepared skillet until golden brown. Fry only a few at a time to stop them from sticking.

16. Serve with cauliflower rice or coconut aminos for dipping.

Roast with Brussel Sprouts

You will be using a slow cooker. Yes, this on the test list because things get overcooked in them. As long as you watch your meat they are a great tool to use.

Ingredients for Meat

- 1 ½ Tbsp. apple cider vinegar

- 3 Tbsp. butter, grass-fed

- 2 Tbsp. XCT oil

- 1 Tsp. dried oregano

- 1 Tbsp. turmeric, ground

- 2 Tbsp. Himalayan pink sea salt

- 1 lb. skirt steak or bottom sirloin, grass-fed

Ingredients for Brussel sprouts

- 2 tsp. turmeric, ground

- 2 tsp. Himalayan pink sea salt

- 2 Tbsp. butter, grass-fed

- 1 lb. Brussel sprouts, halved

Directions for meat

1. Coat meat with oregano, turmeric, and salt.

2. Put meat into the slow cooker.

3. Pour XCT oil over meat. Mix in butter.

4. Set slow cooker to low and cook for 6 to 8 hours or until meat can be shredded with two forks.

5. Once meat is shredded and the vinegar and stir.

Directions for Brussel sprouts

1. Heat oven to 300.

2. Put sprouts in a buttered baking pan

3. Sprinkle with turmeric and salt.

4. Bake 30 to 45 minutes.

Salad with Rosemary Vinaigrette and Chocolate Drizzled Pears

Ingredients for Salad

- 1 small sliced shallot

- 3 cups organic baby greens

Toss together in bowl and set to the side.

Ingredients for the Rosemary Lemon Vinaigrette

- Freshly ground pepper

- Pinch Himalayan pink sea salt

- 1 ¼-inch slice of peeled pear

- 1/8 tsp. Dijon mustard

- 1 Tbsp. fresh rosemary, chopped

- 1 clove garlic, crushed

- ½ cup XCT oil

- Juice of half a lemon

Blend ingredients until smooth. Set to the side.

Ingredients for Chocolate Pear Drizzle

- ¼ cup goat cheese, crumbled

- ¼ tsp. fresh rosemary, chopped fine

- 1 to 2 pinches cayenne pepper

- ½ oz. chocolate

- 1 Tbsp. fresh thyme, chopped

- 1 tsp. raw, organic honey

- 1 sliced pear with skins on

Directions

1. Heat oven to 350. Put parchment paper on cookie sheet. Put pears out on a baking sheet. Drizzle thyme and honey. Bake until soft, about 8 to 10 minutes.

2. While pears are in the oven, melt chocolate in a pot on medium heat. Once melted, add rosemary and cayenne pepper, stir well. Set aside.

3. Once pears are done, take them out of the oven. Spoon the chocolate sauce over the pears. Set to the side.

4. Once you are ready to serve the salad. Toss the salad with vinaigrette. Put the goat cheese and pears on top.

5. Serve and enjoy.

Hanger Steak with Herb Butter

Ingredients

- 3 cups spinach

- Pinch Himalayan pink sea salt

- 2 Tbsp. mixed herbs, chopped (rosemary, thyme, oregano)

- 1 Tbsp. chives, minced

- 4 Tbsp. butter, unsalted, grass-fed, room temperature

- 1 lemon

- 1 Tbsp. Brain Octane oil

- ½ lb. hanger steak

Directions

1. Rub steak with Brain Octane oil. Set to the side.

2. Grate 2 tsp. zest off the lemon. Cut the lemon into wedges. Squeeze 1 tsp. lemon juice. Put the wedges to the side.

3. In small bowl, mix 1 tsp. salt, herbs, chives, butter, and zest. Stir in lemon juice. Mix well to combine.

4. Place grill pan over medium-high heat. Or you could fire up your grill. Season steak with salt. Place on grill pan and reduce to medium-low. Do not char the meat. Cook 5 to 7 minutes each side for rare, 6 to 7 minutes each side for medium-rare. Transfer steak to plate.

Place 2 ½ Tbsp. butter on top and let rest for about 5 minutes.

5. Save remaining butter for use another time.

6. Slice steak across the grain, thinly.

7. Serve with spinach. Top spinach with meat juices and lemon juice.

8. Enjoy!

Dessert Recipes

Chocolate Cupcakes

Ingredients

- 1 Tbsp. sweet rice flour

- Chocolate powder

- 1 tsp. cocoa powder

- 2 tsp. mold-free, lab-tested vanilla powder

- 6 large eggs, separated, room temperature

- Pinch pink Himalayan salt

- 6 oz. or 1 ½ sticks unsalted, grass-fed butter, room temperature

- 12 oz. dark chocolate chips (make sure 85% cacao)

- 6 Tbsp. xylitol

- 6 Tbsp. erythritol

Directions

1. Heat oven to 350. Place racks in the lower and upper third of oven. Line 2 muffin tins with cupcake liners.

2. Pulse erythritol and zylitol in blender until ground finely. Set to the side.

3. Bring 2 cups water to a simmer in small pot on medium-low heat.

4. Put chocolate and butter in heatproof bowl that will sit on the saucepan but not touching water. Place bowl on pan and stir until butter and chocolate are melted. This should take about 10 minutes.

5. Take off the heat and set to the side to cool.

6. In stand mixer with paddle attachment, beat 6 Tbsp. of the xylitol/erythritol, salt, egg yolks on medium-high until mixture is pale and thick. This should take about 3 minutes. Fold the egg mixture into the chocolate and stir in rice flour, cocoa powder, and vanilla powder.

7. Using an electric mixer, in different bowl, beat egg whites until soft peaks form

8. Slowly beat in the xylitol/erythritol, increase speed to medium-high and continue to beat until medium peaks form.

9. Gently fold the egg mixture into the chocolate mixture, about 1/3 at a time, until combined. Put ¼ cup batter into each of the cupcake papers. You will probably only use 20.

10. Bake about 25 minutes or a toothpick inserted come out with a couple moist crumbs.

11. Let cool about 5 minutes before putting on a cooling rack. Let cool completely.

Ice Cream

Ingredients

- 5 ½ Tbsp. or 80 grams erythritol or xylitol – you can add up to 160 grams

- 3 Tbsp. + 2 tsp. or 50 grams XCT oil – must use for consistency

- 7 Tbsp. or 100 grams coconut oil

- 7 Tbsp. or 100 grams butter, grass-fed

- 1-gram Vitamin C – ascorbic acid or 10 drops lime juice or apple cider vinegar to taste

- 2 tsp. vanilla powder

- 4 yolks + 4 whole eggs

- 100 grams – less than ½ cup water or ice; add less than you might need, and increase as you need it.

Directions

1. Put all ingredients but the ice/water in blender. Blend until butter is creamy. This take a little while.

2. Add either the water or ice and blend again until well mixed. If you want creamy ice cream, blend to a yogurt consistency. If you like an icier, firmer texture, add more ice or water.

3. Put into the ice cream maker. Follow the manufacturer's instructions for ice cream.

*You can be as creative here as you want. You could add organic frozen strawberries, or other favorite fruit, or even low-toxin chocolate powder. Just add to blender while mixing the other ingredients.

Coconut Berry Bites

Ingredients

- ¼ cup organic goji berries

- ½ cup freshly grated coconut

- ½ cup raw honey organic

- 1 cup chocolate powder, organic

- 1 cup organic, raw cacao butter

Directions

1. Place the cacao butter into a double boiler and melt it.

2. Add the honey, stir until everything is melted.

3. Add chocolate powder, again stir until everything is smooth.

4. Add the goji berries and coconut, mix well.

5. Pour into any mold – an ice cube tray would be good to use.

6. Place in fridge until hard.

7. Enjoy!

Chocolate Cups

Ingredients

- 2 packets Stevia
- ½ tsp. Vanillamax
- ¾ cup chocolate powder
- 1 cup cacao butter
- Raw nuts of choice

Directions

1. Place cacao butter into double boiler and melt until liquid.

2. Put stevia, vanillamax, and chocolate powder in bowl.

3. Add the melted cacao butter slowly to dry mix. Stir until no longer lumpy.

4. In a muffin pan, place cupcake papers, put nuts of choice.

5. Pour chocolate mixture over nuts filling them about ¼ up.

6. Place in fridge to harden.

7. Enjoy!

Pumpkin Pie

Ingredients

- 5 Tbsp. of Collagelatin that's been dissolved in 1/3 cup boiling water

- ½ tsp. sea salt

- 2 heaping tsp. cinnamon

- 2 tsp. pumpkin spice or make your own (recipe follows)

- 1 tsp. VanillaMax

- 1/3 cup xylitol

- 1 cup coconut milk

- 2 egg yolks

- ¼ cup butter, grass-fed

- 5 Tbsp. Brain Octane Oil

- 2 cups pumpkin, steamed or sweet potato, warmed

Directions

1. Place all of the ingredients in a blender and blend until everything is creamy.

2. If you would like a crust, mix sweet potato or almond flour with salt and enough butter to keep the dough together. Add cold water if it isn't sticking together. Press the crust into pie pan.

3. Pour filling over crust, or into pie pan, if you don't want a crust. Chill pie in freezer at least an hour or place in the refrigerator overnight.

4. To make it extra special, put some whipped coconut cream on top with a dust of cinnamon.

Pumpkin Pie Spice

Ingredients

- ¼ cup cinnamon

- 4 tsp. nutmeg

- 4 tsp. ginger

- 2 tsp. ground allspice

Directions

Mix well and store in an airtight container.

Coffee Cupcakes

Ingredients

- 1 Tbsp. sweet rice flour – has to be sweet the normal rice flour is gritty – omit if don't have

- 1 tsp. very fine ground coffee beans

- 1 tsp. vanilla powder

- 6 room temperature eggs, separated

- Small pinch Himalayan pink sea salt

- 3/4 cup butter, grass-fed, room temperature

- 12 oz. dark chocolate, 85 percent cacao, chips or chopped

- 6 Tbsp. erythritol

- 6 Tbsp. xylitol

Note: You can make a dozen by reducing the recipe by 1/3. If you want or need 2 dozen just increase the recipe by 1/3.

Directions

1. Heat oven to 350

2. Put cupcake liners in 18 muffin tin holes.

3. Put the xylitol and erythritol in blender. Pulse until both are a fine powder. Set to the side.

4. Melt butter and chocolate in heavy pot over low heat. Stir constantly, until it is smooth.

5. Take off the heat. Stir often as it starts to cool. Set aside.

6. Mix 6 egg yolks, salt and 6 Tbsp. of the powdered erythritol/xylitol on medium speed for 3 minutes until mixture turns thick and pale.

7. Gently fold the egg mix into the chocolate, and then add the vanilla, coffee, and floue.

8. In another bowl, beat egg whites until soft peaks form. Slowly add the remaining 6 Tbsp. of erythritol/xylitol and continue to beat until medium peaks form. Fold everything together and little at a time until all incorporated.

9. Fill cupcake lines ¾ full. Bake 11 minutes. Rotate pan and bake for 11 minutes more.

10. Cool on wire rack completely.

11. If you would like to frost them, you can make a frosting by mixing a sweetener of your choice, butter, cocoa powder, and vanilla together.

12. Enjoy!

Blueberry Gelato

Ingredients

- 2 grams ascorbic acid

- 3 Tbsp. xylitol

- Pinch of VanillaMax

- 2 free range egg yolks

- 3 Tbsp. Brain Octane oil

- 5 oz. coconut milk

- 10 oz. blueberries, organic, frozen is fine

Directions

1. Put everything in a blender until creamy and smooth.

2. Pour into either a silicone ice cube tray or an ice cream maker. If using ice cube tray, freeze for 3 hours, stir every hour.

3. Once the ice cubes are frozen. Pop them out and put them in your blender. Blend briefly until smooth.

4. Enjoy!

Smoothie Recipes

Green Tea Smoothie

Ingredients

- 10 ice cubes

- ½ cup coconut milk

- 3 Tbsp. collagen peptide

- 3 tsp. xylitol

- 1 avocado

- 2 tsp. butter

- 3 free range egg yolks

- Pinch of matcha or green tea, ground

Directions

Throw everything in a blender and blend on high until everything is smooth.

Strawberry Smoothie

Ingredients

- Handful of ice cubes

- 4 Organic strawberries – frozen is okay

- 1 Tbsp. coconut oil

- ½ avocado

- 2 scoops whey protein powder

Directions

Put everything in the blender and blend until smooth

Chocolate Blueberry Smoothie

Ingredients

- 2 tsp. MCT oil

- 2 Tbsp. grass-fed butter

- ¼ cup blueberries, frozen

- ½ to 1 whole avocado

- 2 scoops chocolate whey protein powder

- 2 eggs

- 1 cup coconut milk

- 12 oz. ice cubes

Directions

Put everything in your blender. Blend on high. You may have to scrape the sides of the blender to incorporate all the powder. Add ice cubes until you have it the consistency you like.

Chocolate Smoothie

Ingredients

- Handful ice cubes

- 1 Tbsp. grass-fed butter

- 2 free range eggs

- 2 scoops whey protein powder

- 1 cup raw milk

- ½ Tbsp. cacao powder

Directions

Put everything in your blender and blend until smooth.

Superfood Smoothie

Ingredients

- 1 scoop chocolate whey protein powder

- ½ Tbsp. cacao powder

- ½ Tbsp. maca

- 1 Tbsp. chia seeds

- ½ cup blueberries frozen

- ½ avocado

- ½ cup kefir

- ½ cup raw milk

Directions

1. Put kefir and milk into blender. Add all other ingredients and blend until smooth.

2. Enjoy!

Spicy Smoothie

Ingredients

- 1 packet of stevia

- Pinch of Himalayan pink sea salt

- ½ tsp. cinnamon

- ¼ tsp. cayenne pepper

- ½ tsp. ginger

- ½ tsp. turmeric

- 1 Tbsp. chia seeds

- ½ cup papaya chunks, frozen or fresh

- ½ cup blueberries, frozen or fresh

- 1 cup room temperature green tea

Directions

Put everything in a blender until smooth

Detox Smoothie

Ingredients

- 1 tsp. ray honey

- 1 cup kale, remove stems

- 1 banana

- ½ lime, seeded and peeled

- ½ lemon, seeded and peeled

- 1 cup filtered water

Directions

Put everything in a blender and blend until smooth.

Goji Berry Super Smoothie

Ingredients

- Pinch Himalayan pink sea salt

- ½ Tbsp. coconut oil

- ½ cup mango slices, frozen

- 2 Tbsp. goji berries

- 1 cup filtered water

Directions

Put everything in a blender and blend until smooth.

Conclusion

Thank you for making it through to the end of *Bulletproof Diet: Eat Fats, Lose Fats*, hope it was informative and able to provide you with the necessary means you require to achieve your goals whatever it may be.

The next step is to take this information and come up with actions for you to become a new and improved version of yourself. These plentiful tips and tricks will help you get on the right track to becoming Bulletproof.

Take the recipes and make them yours. I hope they will help you enjoy the Bulletproof Diet and kick start your body's fat burning engine. There is a variety of different foods included in the recipes. I hope you will find something to your liking. I particularly enjoyed having the dessert recipes included. Most health diets do not let you eat sweets thus this is an added sweet bonus.

Please feel free to make the recipes work for you. There are different fruits you could switch out in the smoothies. So, change it up for your taste and preference.

Again, thank you for purchasing this book.

Finally, if you found this book useful in anyway, a review on Amazon is always appreciated!

www.ingramcontent.com/pod-product-compliance
Lightning Source LLC
Chambersburg PA
CBHW060152290526
45789CB00003B/1005